This log belongs to:

____

Date Started:

____

Date Ended:

____

Week Starting:

Write down the blood sugar level in each box, use a highlighter if another illness occurred that day.

	AM	PM
Sunday		
Monday		
Tuesday		
Wednesday		
Thursday		
Friday		
Saturday		

Week Starting:

Write down the blood sugar level in each box, use a highlighter if another illness occurred that day.

	AM	PM
Sunday		
Monday		
Tuesday		
Wednesday		
Thursday		
Friday		
Saturday		

Week Starting:

Write down the blood sugar level in each box, use a highlighter if another illness occurred that day.

	AM	PM
Sunday		
Monday		
Tuesday		
Wednesday		
Thursday		
Friday		
Saturday		

Week Starting:

Write down the blood sugar level in each box, use a highlighter if another illness occurred that day.

	AM	PM
Sunday		
Monday		
Tuesday		
Wednesday		
Thursday		
Friday		
Saturday		

Week Starting:

Write down the blood sugar level in each box, use a highlighter if another illness occurred that day.

	AM	PM
Sunday		
Monday		
Tuesday		
Wednesday		
Thursday		
Friday		
Saturday		

Week Starting:

Write down the blood sugar level in each box, use a highlighter if another illness occurred that day.

	AM	PM
Sunday		
Monday		
Tuesday		
Wednesday		
Thursday		
Friday		
Saturday		

Week Starting:

Write down the blood sugar level in each box, use a highlighter if another illness occurred that day.

	AM	PM
Sunday		
Monday		
Tuesday		
Wednesday		
Thursday		
Friday		
Saturday		

Week Starting:

Write down the blood sugar level in each box, use a highlighter if another illness occurred that day.

	AM	PM
Sunday		
Monday		
Tuesday		
Wednesday		
Thursday		
Friday		
Saturday		

Week Starting:

Write down the blood sugar level in each box, use a highlighter if another illness occurred that day.

	AM	PM
Sunday		
Monday		
Tuesday		
Wednesday		
Thursday		
Friday		
Saturday		

Week Starting:

Write down the blood sugar level in each box, use a highlighter if another illness occurred that day.

	AM	PM
Sunday		
Monday		
Tuesday		
Wednesday		
Thursday		
Friday		
Saturday		

Week Starting:

Write down the blood sugar level in each box, use a highlighter if another illness occurred that day.

	AM	PM
Sunday		
Monday		
Tuesday		
Wednesday		
Thursday		
Friday		
Saturday		

Week Starting:

Write down the blood sugar level in each box, use a highlighter if another illness occurred that day.

	AM	PM
Sunday		
Monday		
Tuesday		
Wednesday		
Thursday		
Friday		
Saturday		

Week Starting:

Write down the blood sugar level in each box, use a highlighter if another illness occurred that day.

	AM	PM
Sunday		
Monday		
Tuesday		
Wednesday		
Thursday		
Friday		
Saturday		

Week Starting:

Write down the blood sugar level in each box, use a highlighter if another illness occurred that day.

	AM	PM
Sunday		
Monday		
Tuesday		
Wednesday		
Thursday		
Friday		
Saturday		

Week Starting:

Write down the blood sugar level in each box, use a highlighter if another illness occurred that day.

	AM	PM
Sunday		
Monday		
Tuesday		
Wednesday		
Thursday		
Friday		
Saturday		

Week Starting:

Write down the blood sugar level in each box, use a highlighter if another illness occurred that day.

	AM	PM
Sunday		
Monday		
Tuesday		
Wednesday		
Thursday		
Friday		
Saturday		

Week Starting:

Write down the blood sugar level in each box, use a highlighter if another illness occurred that day.

	AM	PM
Sunday		
Monday		
Tuesday		
Wednesday		
Thursday		
Friday		
Saturday		

Week Starting:

Write down the blood sugar level in each box, use a highlighter if another illness occurred that day.

	AM	PM
Sunday		
Monday		
Tuesday		
Wednesday		
Thursday		
Friday		
Saturday		

Week Starting:

Write down the blood sugar level in each box, use a highlighter if another illness occurred that day.

	AM	PM
Sunday		
Monday		
Tuesday		
Wednesday		
Thursday		
Friday		
Saturday		

Week Starting:

Write down the blood sugar level in each box, use a highlighter if another illness occurred that day.

	AM	PM
Sunday		
Monday		
Tuesday		
Wednesday		
Thursday		
Friday		
Saturday		

Week Starting:

Write down the blood sugar level in each box, use a highlighter if another illness occurred that day.

	AM	PM
Sunday		
Monday		
Tuesday		
Wednesday		
Thursday		
Friday		
Saturday		

Week Starting:

Write down the blood sugar level in each box, use a highlighter if another illness occurred that day.

	AM	PM
Sunday		
Monday		
Tuesday		
Wednesday		
Thursday		
Friday		
Saturday		

Week Starting:

Write down the blood sugar level in each box, use a highlighter if another illness occurred that day.

	AM	PM
Sunday		
Monday		
Tuesday		
Wednesday		
Thursday		
Friday		
Saturday		

Week Starting:

Write down the blood sugar level in each box, use a highlighter if another illness occurred that day.

	AM	PM
Sunday		
Monday		
Tuesday		
Wednesday		
Thursday		
Friday		
Saturday		

Week Starting:

Write down the blood sugar level in each box, use a highlighter if another illness occurred that day.

	AM	PM
Sunday		
Monday		
Tuesday		
Wednesday		
Thursday		
Friday		
Saturday		

Week Starting:

Write down the blood sugar level in each box, use a highlighter if another illness occurred that day.

	AM	PM
Sunday		
Monday		
Tuesday		
Wednesday		
Thursday		
Friday		
Saturday		

Week Starting:

Write down the blood sugar level in each box, use a highlighter if another illness occurred that day.

	AM	PM
Sunday		
Monday		
Tuesday		
Wednesday		
Thursday		
Friday		
Saturday		

Week Starting:

Write down the blood sugar level in each box, use a highlighter if another illness occurred that day.

	AM	PM
Sunday		
Monday		
Tuesday		
Wednesday		
Thursday		
Friday		
Saturday		

Week Starting:

Write down the blood sugar level in each box, use a highlighter if another illness occurred that day.

	AM	PM
Sunday		
Monday		
Tuesday		
Wednesday		
Thursday		
Friday		
Saturday		

Week Starting:

Write down the blood sugar level in each box, use a highlighter if another illness occurred that day.

	AM	PM
Sunday		
Monday		
Tuesday		
Wednesday		
Thursday		
Friday		
Saturday		

Week Starting:

Write down the blood sugar level in each box, use a highlighter if another illness occurred that day.

	AM	PM
Sunday		
Monday		
Tuesday		
Wednesday		
Thursday		
Friday		
Saturday		

Week Starting:

Write down the blood sugar level in each box, use a highlighter if another illness occurred that day.

	AM	PM
Sunday		
Monday		
Tuesday		
Wednesday		
Thursday		
Friday		
Saturday		

Week Starting:

Write down the blood sugar level in each box, use a highlighter if another illness occurred that day.

	AM	PM
Sunday		
Monday		
Tuesday		
Wednesday		
Thursday		
Friday		
Saturday		

Week Starting:

Write down the blood sugar level in each box, use a highlighter if another illness occurred that day.

	AM	PM
Sunday		
Monday		
Tuesday		
Wednesday		
Thursday		
Friday		
Saturday		

Week Starting:

Write down the blood sugar level in each box, use a highlighter if another illness occurred that day.

	AM	PM
Sunday		
Monday		
Tuesday		
Wednesday		
Thursday		
Friday		
Saturday		

Week Starting:

Write down the blood sugar level in each box, use a highlighter if another illness occurred that day.

	AM	PM
Sunday		
Monday		
Tuesday		
Wednesday		
Thursday		
Friday		
Saturday		

Week Starting:

Write down the blood sugar level in each box, use a highlighter if another illness occurred that day.

	AM	PM
Sunday		
Monday		
Tuesday		
Wednesday		
Thursday		
Friday		
Saturday		

Week Starting:

Write down the blood sugar level in each box, use a highlighter if another illness occurred that day.

	AM	PM
Sunday		
Monday		
Tuesday		
Wednesday		
Thursday		
Friday		
Saturday		

Week Starting:

Write down the blood sugar level in each box, use a highlighter if another illness occurred that day.

	AM	PM
Sunday		
Monday		
Tuesday		
Wednesday		
Thursday		
Friday		
Saturday		

Week Starting:

Write down the blood sugar level in each box, use a highlighter if another illness occurred that day.

	AM	PM
Sunday		
Monday		
Tuesday		
Wednesday		
Thursday		
Friday		
Saturday		

Week Starting:

Write down the blood sugar level in each box, use a highlighter if another illness occurred that day.

	AM	PM
Sunday		
Monday		
Tuesday		
Wednesday		
Thursday		
Friday		
Saturday		

Week Starting:

Write down the blood sugar level in each box, use a highlighter if another illness occurred that day.

	AM	PM
Sunday		
Monday		
Tuesday		
Wednesday		
Thursday		
Friday		
Saturday		

Week Starting:

Write down the blood sugar level in each box, use a highlighter if another illness occurred that day.

	AM	PM
Sunday		
Monday		
Tuesday		
Wednesday		
Thursday		
Friday		
Saturday		

Week Starting:

Write down the blood sugar level in each box, use a highlighter if another illness occurred that day.

	AM	PM
Sunday		
Monday		
Tuesday		
Wednesday		
Thursday		
Friday		
Saturday		

Week Starting:

Write down the blood sugar level in each box, use a highlighter if another illness occurred that day.

	AM	PM
Sunday		
Monday		
Tuesday		
Wednesday		
Thursday		
Friday		
Saturday		

Week Starting:

Write down the blood sugar level in each box, use a highlighter if another illness occurred that day.

	AM	PM
Sunday		
Monday		
Tuesday		
Wednesday		
Thursday		
Friday		
Saturday		

Week Starting:

Write down the blood sugar level in each box, use a highlighter if another illness occurred that day.

	AM	PM
Sunday		
Monday		
Tuesday		
Wednesday		
Thursday		
Friday		
Saturday		

Week Starting:

Write down the blood sugar level in each box, use a highlighter if another illness occurred that day.

	AM	PM
Sunday		
Monday		
Tuesday		
Wednesday		
Thursday		
Friday		
Saturday		

Week Starting:

Write down the blood sugar level in each box, use a highlighter if another illness occurred that day.

	AM	PM
Sunday		
Monday		
Tuesday		
Wednesday		
Thursday		
Friday		
Saturday		

Week Starting:

Write down the blood sugar level in each box, use a highlighter if another illness occurred that day.

	AM	PM
Sunday		
Monday		
Tuesday		
Wednesday		
Thursday		
Friday		
Saturday		

Week Starting:

Write down the blood sugar level in each box, use a highlighter if another illness occurred that day.

	AM	PM
Sunday		
Monday		
Tuesday		
Wednesday		
Thursday		
Friday		
Saturday		

Week Starting:

Write down the blood sugar level in each box, use a highlighter if another illness occurred that day.

	AM	PM
Sunday		
Monday		
Tuesday		
Wednesday		
Thursday		
Friday		
Saturday